101 Natural Hair Care Tips for Curly, Kinky & Coily Hair

Get ShidaNaturalized!

By

RASHIDA 'SHIDANATURAL' GODBOLD

ISBN-9798634039411

Alicia Dunams,

Without you, this book would be non-existent. Your "Bestseller in a Weekend" course is what I needed to get this book written and published. Thank you for being my accountability partner / coach and helping me get it done!

To my readers: If you are thinking about writing a book, contact Alicia Dunams to help you get started and complete your book in record time! alicia@aliciadunams.com

To My Family,

A special heartfelt thanks goes out to you for being my guinea pigs as I tested new formulas for the ShidaNatural's Healthy Hair Care Products line. I also want to thank you for the many years of doing EXACTLY what I tell you to do to your hair as research for the content I put together for this book.

Love you always!

Contents

Acknowledgements

This book is dedicated to all my Natural / Curly Girls (and Guys) who strive to make every day a Happy Hair Day!

I'd like to thank everyone who supported me by purchasing this book; purchasing my hair products; being a client at KinHairitage Natural Hair Salon; subscribing to my YouTube channel; and trusting me to help you with your natural curly, kinky and coily hair challenges.

With the purchase of this book, you get this product for FREE!

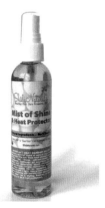

ShidaNatural's Mist of Shine & Heat Protector contains oil of safflower, which protects the hair from heat without causing buildup on the hair like silicone-based heat protectants. Safflower oil also nourishes hair follicles and stimulates blood circulation to promote thicker, longer, shinier hair. Specially formulated with essential oils for an appealing, natural fragrance and a light, non-greasy feel. Hair of all types and textures will benefit from this oil mist.

To get your FREE bottle:

Go to www.ShidaNaturals.com

Add ShidaNatural's Mist of Shine to cart

Checkout with discount code, **101TIPS**

Introduction

As a fellow naturalista or naturalisto, you've probably heard of the letter/number hair typing system. This hair typing system describes the different shapes of hair strands. You know— 3a, 3b, 4a, 4c, etc. Many of you may use this hair typing system. The problem I personally have with these classifications is that they do not evaluate texture, density, length, and porosity. It only evaluates the shape of the hair strand; Straight, Wavy, Loose S-shape Curl, Tight S-shape Curl, Coily/Corkscrew, Kinky, etc.

My hair salon clients and others with whom I communicate frequently ask me to identify their hair type using the letter/number hair typing system so they can make decisions about their hair, such as choosing which products they need for their hair or how they should style. Rather than give them a short "You are a 4a hair texture" answer, I look at the shape of their hair strands, or CURL PATTERN; how fine, medium, or coarse their hair strands are, or their TEXTURE; how many hair strands they have on their head, or hair DENSITY; how much moisture their hair absorbs and retains or POROSITY. I then ask if their hair is always dry, and if they normally have a dry or itchy scalp. All these things must be considered when choosing what products/ingredients to use (or not use), hairstyles, product application techniques, how to manipulate your hair, how frequently you should cleanse and condition your hair, and how you maintain your hairstyle.

If, after reading this introduction, you are excited and yearn to learn much, much more...
Keep reading!

"Learn about your hair today so you can love it tomorrow!"

1

Cleansing

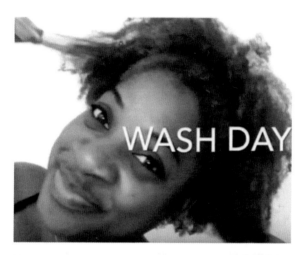

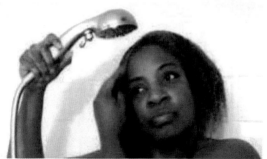

*Still photos taken from an actual YouTube tutorial video
of ShidaNatural cleansing her hair
www.youtube.com/shidanatural*

How to Cleanse

First start with a warm water rinse (in the shower for best results) to open the hair cuticles and remove the topical dirt and debris. Cleanse the scalp first by getting underneath the hair and massaging your cleansing product into the scalp with the cushions of your fingertips. Take advantage of this time to give yourself a scalp massage, which increases blood flow and stimulates the follicles, all of which makes hair grow faster. Next, rinse with warm water while allowing the cleansing agent to run down the hair strands without manipulating the hair too much. Then, cleanse the hair strands with your hands and fingers in a smooth-and-rake motion. For best styling results, rake and smooth the hair strands in the direction in which you will be styling your hair. This method of cleansing the hair and scalp reduces tangles and frizz. Never be vigorous when cleansing your hair, as you will disturb your curl pattern, and make it harder to detangle and style.

What to Cleanse With

There are a variety of different elements you can cleanse your hair with. You can use water, shampoo, conditioner, and a host of other things; it's about your preference. You may consider cleansing your hair and scalp with plain water if you want to save money on hair products (since water is the absolute cheapest hair care product) or want to maintain a chemical-free (or product-free) hair care routine. You may also consider "water-washing" if you want to redistribute and retain your hair's natural oils (sebum) during the cleansing process. The most popular cleansing product that we've grown accustomed to using since we were babies is shampoo! Remember Johnson & Johnson shampoo, either as a kid or as a parent gently cleansing our precious little baby's hair? You may opt to use shampoo as your cleanser if you like that squeaky clean feel, or like to suds up. The cleansing agent in most shampoos (which is called a sulfate) has been known to be a bit harsh as it strips the hair of all its natural oils and moisture causing additional dryness and frizz especially on natural / curly hair. Because of this concern, we have been introduced to other types of shampoos that may not be as drying... particularly sulfate-free shampoo, for one. A popular "no-poo" or shampoo alternative, especially among us naturals / curlies, is Conditioner-Washing. This is when one uses conditioner in place of shampoo or other cleansing product to cleanse their hair and scalp. The "Conditioner Only" method is a great choice if your hair is very thick, dry, tangles very easily, and/or is hard to manage. This has been my personal preference for years since conditioner-washing keeps my hair more moisturized and less tangled and frizzy. Other shampoo alternatives are as follows: apple cider vinegar, baking soda, oil-washing, bentonite clay, castile soap, and dry shampoo just to name a few. Like I said, it's your preference. and your choice should be based on your hair care needs and lifestyle.

Where to Cleanse

It's important to make sure you cleanse your scalp, hairline, and hair strands from root to tip.

What to Cleanse First

Cleanse the scalp and hairline first! The scalp is where dirt, dandruff, debris, oils, excessive sebum, dead skin cells, sweat, bacteria, and product buildup accumulate. A clean scalp and unclogged hair follicles promote a healthy scalp, resulting in healthy hair growth.

What to Cleanse Next

After cleansing the scalp and hairline, work the hair strands from root to tip, manipulating the hair in a smooth and rake motion rather than a circular motion. This method of cleansing forces the hair cuticle to lay down and reduces tangles. With natural hair, the hair cuticle (the outside layer of the hair strand) likes to lift around the bend of each curl, causing hair strands to tangle with one another. When thinking of a hair strand, think of a pinecone. When the pines are lifted on a pinecone, looking and feeling prickly, that's what a hair strand looks like when the cuticle is lifted. When the pines are laying down flat, looking and feeling smooth, that's what a hair strand looks like when the cuticle is laid down.

6

What to Focus on the Most

During the cleansing process, the focus should mostly be on the scalp as it is not as exposed as the hair strands, especially if your hair is thick. Dirt and debris cannot be removed from the scalp as easily as it can from the hair strands.

7

Different Ways to Cleanse

The most common way to cleanse your hair is to pour a desired amount of your cleansing product in the palm of your hand, rub hands together, then lather up the hair in a rigorous, circular motion. That's what we see on TV, right? That may be an effective way for some, but for those of us with natural / curly hair, this way may result in a mangled, tangled mess! If you want to keep your hair controlled and tangle-free during the cleansing process, one effective way would be to cleanse your hair in sections, using the technique in number 1.

How Often You Should Cleanse

How often you cleanse your hair and scalp will depend on numerous factors, including your lifestyle, length of hair, thickness of hair, hair texture, how you style your hair, and the climate you live in. For instance, if you have a short, naturally curly 'do and you work out in the gym a lot, you might cleanse your hair every day. If you wear your hair in protective styles (which will be discussed later in this book) you may cleanse once a week, once a month, or once every couple months. If you wear your natural curls where you apply styling products frequently, you may cleanse your hair every few days or once a week. If you work in an environment where you are around dirt and debris all day long, you may have to cleanse your hair more frequently. Get to know your hair and scalp's needs, and you will know how often you need to cleanse your hair and scalp.

Cleanse versus Wash

The difference between the words cleanse and wash is simple! When you wash something or someone, you use soap or detergent to strip away everything from the surface. For example... We wash our clothes and we wash our car. When you cleanse, you "gently" remove dirt and debris from the surface.

For example, we cleanse our faces and, in getting back to the main topic, our hair. This is why I use the word cleanse instead of wash in this section; I want to stress the importance of being gentle to your hair during the cleaning process, rather than harsh and rigorous.

10

Cleanse versus Shampoo

You may opt to "cleanse" your hair with something other than shampoo. Therefore, if you're not using shampoo to cleanse your hair, then why would you use the verb shampoo? Makes sense?

11

Is Shampoo Bad?

I would not view shampoo as good or bad since the use of shampoo and what kind depends on many factors. Your shampoo needs are determined by your hair's texture, your hair's condition, your hair care routine, how often you cleanse your hair, whether or not you color your hair, if your hair is extra oily, if your hair is extra dry, etc. Some shampoos may be harsher than others. An alternative to traditional shampoo is a sulfate-free shampoo which may not be as harsh or drying.

12

Natural Shampoo Alternatives

We briefly discussed shampoo alternatives in "What to Cleanse With;" but, for those who prefer to use all natural products, here are some "natural" shampoo alternatives:

- Water – You can't get any more natural than water! If you are considering using only water to wash your hair, it is recommended that you install a shower filter, which will soften hard water and remove the chemicals from your shower water. Another tip would be to use warm water to open the cuticle and dissolve debris, and cool water to close the hair cuticle to seal in moisture and have shinier hair.

- Apple Cider Vinegar – Probably the most popular shampoo alternative, especially amongst the natural hair community, apple cider vinegar's acidic properties balance the scalp's PH, which can be very beneficial if you have excessively oily hair and scalp. This shampoo alternative also does a good job clarifying the hair and removing product build up, resulting in shiny hair.

- Baking Soda – Baking soda can not only be used to clarify the hair, but also to exfoliate the scalp and give a deep cleansing of the hair follicles.

- Ayurvedic Powders – A unique shampoo alternative derived from India, Skikaki and Aritha Ayurvedic powders act as natural cleansers. Shikaki is known to strengthen hair roots and cure dandruff while Aritha powder (also called Reetha or Soapnut) acts as a natural shampoo that gives the hair a natural shine.

13

Cleanse Hair in the Shower

Of course it's your preference where you cleanse your hair, but I have found that cleansing your hair in the shower has the most benefits. Cleansing your hair in the shower is probably more comfortable than cleansing while bent over the sink or sitting in the bathtub, because the shower gives you more control when it comes to rinsing. The shower's water, which runs in a downward motion, not only makes detangling easier, but also allows your hair strands to naturally fall in any direction you decide to style your hair, whether to the back, front, side. A handheld shower-head, especially one with stream settings, will aid in a more thorough cleansing, especially on the scalp.

14

What Are Sulfates?

A sulfate is the cleansing agent that produces suds in cleaning products like detergents and shampoos. Sulfates do a great job stripping away dirt and making things like pots, pans, and drinking glasses sparkle, but when it comes to stripping the hair, that may not be so good especially for natural / curly hair.

15

Why is Stripping Bad for Hair?

Natural Curly, Kinky and Coily hair is already naturally dry, thirsty and craves moisture. When using products that strip the hair, you are essentially stripping away EVERYTHING from your hair strands, including your hair's natural oils and moisture.

16

Is that Squeaky Clean sound Good or Bad?

Depending on how active your sebaceous glands are, that "squeaky" clean sound (heard when cleansing the hair) could be good or bad. If you have overactive sebaceous glands, it is very likely that you produce a lot of sebum, which is the natural oil that comes out of your scalp to provide natural moisture and shine to the hair. That extra sebum may result in very oily hair and, if this is the case, you may desire to strip all the oil from your hair and hear that squeaky clean sound, since it's likely you will produce more sebum rapidly. The opposite holds true for someone who may not produce a lot of sebum, or for whom the hair strands are extremely curly, and the sebum doesn't get to the ends of the hair strands that quickly. In this case, you may not want to strip the oil that is in the hair, so you definitely don't want to hear that sound, because that means you stripped every bit of moisture and oil that was keeping your hair healthy, and it could take days to replenish that moisture level.

17

What is a Water Wash?

A water wash is just like it sounds... Cleansing the hair with water only. See tip number 12 for more on water washing.

18

What is a "Pre-Poo?"

Preparing your hair before shampooing can combat the drying effect and tangles that shampoo may contribute to on natural / curly hair. Hot oil treatment, conditioning before shampooing, and detangling are few ways you can pre-poo or prepare your hair before shampooing.

19

How Do You Pre-Poo?

There are many different ways to pre-poo, but I will introduce you to a few simple ways. You can detangle your hair while it's dry by smoothing and raking your fingers through your hair to remove tangles and knots, smoothing the hair cuticle to reduce the number of tangles you may get during the shampoo process. You can do the same thing with conditioner or hot oil for easier detangling and utilize a wide tooth comb, paddle brush, or Denman brush to assist with removing shed hair before shampooing

2

Conditioning

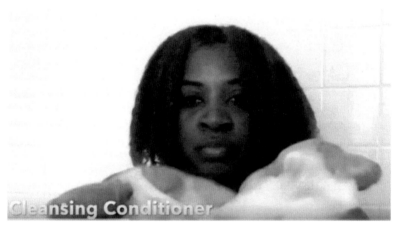

Still photo taken from an actual YouTube tutorial video
of ShidaNatural conditioning her hair
www.youtube.com/shidanatural

20

Why is Conditioning Important?

Conditioning does just like the word says... gets the hair, particularly natural / curly hair, in good or better condition. Conditioning is important to help with moisture, provide control, and prevent frizz resulting in better curl definition and avoid breakage. All of this ultimately results in retaining length while the hair grows.

21

How do You Condition?

The most practical way of conditioning the hair is squeezing, pouring, or pumping your conditioner of choice into the palm of your hair. Don't always go by the amount in the directions, because your hair may require more or less depending on your hair's thickness and density. Rub hands together to emulsify the product, followed by smoothing and raking the conditioner into the hair strands in the direction in which you will be styling your hair. This is the best time to take advantage of an easy detangling opportunity using your fingers, wide-tooth comb, paddle brush, or Denman brush starting with the ends of the hair then working up.

22

What are the Best Conditioners?

The ideal conditioner for natural / curly hair, especially the thick kind, is one that provides a ton of slip; meaning a conditioner that is formulated to make detangling a breeze. A good conditioner is also one that doesn't contain ingredients known to cause a lot of buildup on the hair... and most importantly, it's one that moisturizes the hair.

23

Why are There So Many Conditioners to Choose From?

Why are there so many different kinds of potato chips to choose from? Or cars, or trucks... the list goes on and on! People like variety, and businesses like to offer a lot of different varieties so they can make more money. On the other end of the spectrum, there are different types of conditioners that serve different purposes. You have your rinse-out conditioners and your leave-in conditioners. There are certain conditioners recommended for co-washing. There are others used for detangling, moisturizing, clarifying, and deep conditioning. There are protein-rich conditioners, and let's not forget those conditioners meant to provide protection for color-treated hair. Some conditioners are specially formulated for different hair textures, such as fine, medium, or coarse.

24

Can You Use Only Conditioner to Cleanse Hair?

You may have heard of the conditioner-only method, where you only use conditioner to cleanse your hair and scalp. Many people with natural / curly hair opt for this method of cleansing their hair to avoid the tangles and dryness that sometimes result from using shampoo. This method of cleansing the hair is known as conditioner-washing, or co-washing, for short. More on Co-washing in tip number 27.

25

Do You Always Have to Rinse Out Conditioner?

It is safe and, for most, extremely beneficial to leave some conditioner in your hair, despite the bottle's instructions to rinse completely. Leaving a little conditioner in your hair allows for easier styling with less tangles and frizz. It is suggested, however, that you make sure all the conditioner is rinsed from the scalp to avoid product build-up there.

26

What Ingredients in Conditioners Offer Slip for Easy Combing/Brushing?

'Slip' is a term used to identify a characteristic in a conditioner or other hair product that makes it easier to comb, brush, finger-comb, or otherwise remove tangles and knots from the hair. Finding a conditioner that offers lots of slip is crucial, especially for those with thick, coarse, or unruly natural / curly hair. Some ingredients that are known to provide the best slip are: fatty alcohols such as stearyl alcohol, cetyl alcohol, and cetearyl alcohol; vegetable oils such as olive oil and coconut oil; and butters, such as shea and cocoa butters. We will expand more on these ingredients later on in the book.

27

What is Co-Washing?

Co-washing is short for "conditioner-washing," and means just that; washing the hair and scalp with conditioner only. Some also call it the Conditioner Only Method, as explained in tip number 24.

28

Why is Conditioner More Important than Shampoo?

Sure, it's important to have clean hair; but, for most people, it's even more important to have tangle-free and manageable hair, not to mention those days us curly girls want more definition and shine. The easiest way to achieve those results is with a good conditioner. The majority of shampoos tend to lift the hair strand's outer layer (called the cuticle) resulting in frizz, tangles, and dull-looking hair. Most conditioners do the complete opposite! They smooth down the cuticle, reducing frizz and tangles. This results in curl definition, sleekness, and shine. Let's compare your hair strand to a pinecone. When the pines of a pinecone are sticking out, that's like your hair strands when you use shampoo. When the pines are lying flat and the pinecone is shiny, that's like your hair strands when you use conditioner. The reason your hair shines more when the cuticle, the hair strand's outside layer, is laid down (or flat) is because light can only reflect on a flat surface. Don't you remember learning that in science class!

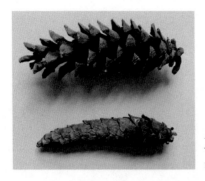

Photo is a pinecone illustration to compare what a hair strand looks like when the cuticle is open versus when it is closed

29

What is "Deep Conditioning?"

Deep conditioning is a personal choice, based on your hair's personal needs. Natural / curly hair that is usually dry and thirsty needs extra moisture and deeper conditioning. Deep conditioning is the act of saturating the hair with moisture, strands past the cuticle (outside layer) to the cortex (middle layer) all the way through to the medulla (inside layer) resulting in softer, more moisturized, healthier-looking hair. <u>Note:</u> You may need to alternate between Moisturizing & Protein Deep Conditions to keep that moisture/protein balance. Both too much moisture and too much protein can cause breakage.

30

How Often Should you Deep Condition?

As stated in tip number 29, deep conditioning is a personal choice based on personal need. Depending on your hair's need, your lifestyle, the climate around you, how you style your hair, and other factors, you can choose to deep condition every day, once a week, once every two weeks, once a month, once every two months, once every six months. It's your choice!

31

How Long Should You Deep Condition For?

This is also your choice, depending on need, how much time you have, and other factors mentioned above. Some leave their deep conditioner on for as little as 15 minutes. Others may leave their deep conditioner anywhere from 2 hours to as long as overnight!

32

What are Different Ways to Deep Condition?

There are 3 basic ways to deep condition and, again, it's your choice which one you choose.

1. Mild Deep Condition: the most practical way to deep condition involves leaving your deep conditioner on your hair (with your hair uncovered), while you shower, for a light deep condition.

2. Moderate Deep Condition: if you want the deep conditioner to penetrate a little deeper into the hair shaft, you can cover your hair with a plastic cap after applying the conditioner to hair that has been rinsed with very warm

water. The steam from the warm water will open up the hair cuticle for a mild penetration of the conditioner into the hair shaft.

3. Intense Deep Condition: for the deepest penetrating version, add some heat or make your own steam. Most hair salons offer these types of deep conditioning treatments. Going under a hooded dryer or a steamer allows the conditioner to get deep into the hair strands leaving you with the softest, moisturized, healthiest-looking hair. You can get these same salon treatments in the comfort of your own home by purchasing a hooded dryer, or a steamer made for home-use!

33

What are Silicones?

Silicones are ingredients added to certain hair products, particularly in conditioners and heat styling hair products, to act as a heat protectant, smooth hair strands, and/or give the hair a sleeker appearance. You can identify silicones, when reading the ingredients list on the label of a hair product by the words cone, conol, or xane in the ingredient name. More on types of silicones in the ingredients chapter.

34

Are Silicones Bad?

Silicones don't necessarily have to be bad for the hair. They can actually benefit the hair by closing the hair's cuticle and sealing split ends to prevent breakage. However, depending on your hair's texture or type, silicones may improve the hair's appearance for some, but not for all. For others, moderate or excessive use of silicones may yield not-so-desired results and can even cause dryness and/or dullness to the hair.

35

Are Expensive Conditioners the Best?

The best conditioners do not have to cost you an arm and a leg. In fact, the conditioners I've been using for years cost me less than $3 and are made of natural, botanical ingredients! More often than not, you're not so much paying for what's in the actual product more than you are the name. It's just like bags... Although Michael Kors and Louis Vuitton both make good quality bags and purses, you will pay more for a LV because you are paying for the name.

36

Can I Make My Own Conditioner / Deep Conditioner?

There are tons and tons of concoctions you can make at home using things you already have in your cupboard! All you need are a few simple ingredients of your choice such as: extra virgin olive oil, coconut oil, mayonnaise, eggs, honey, aloe vera, apple cider vinegar, yogurt, banana, etc. You can even add some of the conditioner you have at home to your deep conditioning concoction. Before you select which ingredients you will whip up, first determine if you need a moisturizing deep conditioner, a protein deep conditioner, or both.

37

How Can I Tell if I Need a Moisturizing Conditioner or a Protein Conditioner?

The most apparent way to tell if you need a moisturizing conditioner is if your hair feels and looks dry and brittle. That's just a given! One way to tell if you need protein is if your hair is overly moisturized, or feels mushy. Then, there's the scientific way to determine if you need moisture or protein, and that is the strand test. There are actually two strand tests you can perform. First thing is to grab a few strands of shed hair by running your clenched fingers down a section of hair to pull out a few shed strands. If you don't get any the first time, try a different section.

1. The Stretch Test – Take one of the shed hair strands and wet it with water. Then, with your thumbs and pointer fingers on each side, slowly and gently stretch the hair strand; then gently release the tension. If the hair strand bounces back to its original state, that means you have the proper moisture/protein balance. If it immediately snaps and breaks, you need moisture. If it stays stretched and does not return to its original state, you need protein.

2. The Porosity Test – Place one of the shed hair strands in a glass of water. If the hair strand sinks to the bottom of

the glass, your hair is porous. What does it mean when your hair is porous? It means that it absorbs moisture quickly but also loses moisture quickly because the cuticle is open. This is an indication of a damaged cuticle and low protein. If the hair strand stays afloat on top of the water for a while, your hair is not porous. This means that the cuticle is closed very tightly, and you may need to clarify the hair of product build up then follow up with a moisturizing conditioner to replenish the moisture that was stripped away during the clarifying process. If the hair strand slowly sinks to the middle, your hair is normal, and a regular conditioning (or a moisturizing conditioner, if you prefer) should be fine.

38
What Ingredients Should I Look for in a Conditioner?

We will talk about ingredients in more depth later in the book; therefore, I will briefly touch on a few ingredients you should look for when reading the back of the conditioner label. The ingredients that I will elaborate on in this section are a sampling of ingredients that offer moisture and manageability to natural / curly hair.

1. Good alcohols, such as Cetyl, Stearyl, and Cetearyl are non-drying, fatty alcohols that act as softeners or emollients, making it easier to detangle and more manageable.

2. Oils & butters like shea butter, extra virgin olive oil, and coconut oil are good to look for in your conditioner, as they are natural ingredients that contribute to the overall health of the hair and provide shine to the hair as well. Unlike other oils, extra virgin olive oil and coconut oil are the only oils that actually penetrate into the hair shaft, providing extra conditioning. Shea butter acts as a sealant to close the cuticle, sealing in moisture.

3. Humectants, such as vegetable glycerin, attract moisture from the air, allowing the hair to retain moisture. Depending on your choice or hairstyle, this could be either a good thing or a not-so-good thing. It's great if you're wearing a wash and go style or some other wet style. If you're wearing your natural hair in a set style, or just got it straightened (or heat-styled), humectants may cause the hair strands to swell and frizz, resulting in a more voluminous look (which many of us don't mind). On the contrary, and depending on one's hair type, humectants may have the opposite effect if the climate is dry; the dry air may actually pull moisture out of the hair.

4. Panthenol (Vitamin B5)

   This B vitamin acts quite similar to a protein, except it improves moisture retention as it penetrates the hair shaft. If you have brittle or fine hair, this is a very effective ingredient to look for in your conditioner.

39

What Ingredients Should I Avoid When Looking for a Conditioner?

If your hair is dry or non-porous, you want to avoid frequent use of certain ingredients that may cause additional dryness, block out moisture, or cause product build up. You want to avoid these ingredients all together if you are following up with a leave-in conditioner, or moisturizer after rinsing out your conditioner. The most common of such ingredients are: Silicones, Mineral Oil, Drying alcohols such as SD alcohol, SD alcohol 40, Alcohol denat, Propanol, Propyl alcohol, and Isopropyl alcohol.

40

Why is it Good to Rinse Conditioner out With Cold Water?

A cold water final rinse yields many benefits. Cold water forces the hair's cuticle to close and lay flat, contributing to better curl definition, better styling results, and shine. As explained in tip number 28, light can only reflect on a flat surface, resulting in a glorious shine when the cuticle is flat.

3

Moisturizing

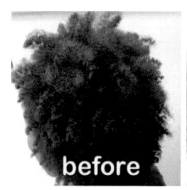
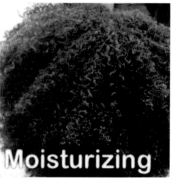
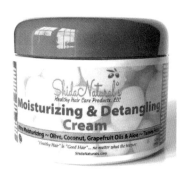
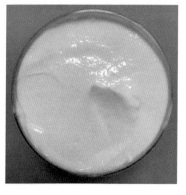

Photos of KinHairitage Salon client's before & after hair that was moisturized with ShidaNatural's Moisturizing & Detangling Cream
www.kinhairitage.com
www.shidanaturals.com

41

What is the Difference Between Moisturizing and Conditioning?

Although there are products that offer both moisturizing and conditioning benefits, there is a difference between the two. As explained in the previous section, the main purpose of conditioner is to help make detangling easier, and the lack of conditioner may cause damage to the hair strands. Conditioner also improves the feel, appearance and manageability of hair and, for those who may get static hair, conditioner reduces static, so hair lays down and you don't look like a porcupine, or like you have a lion's mane! Moisturizing, on the other hand, focuses on moisture levels and maintaining them. The purpose of using a hair moisturizer is to counteract or prevent the hair from feeling hard, dry, and brittle.

42

What Is the Best Moisturizer?

The best moisturizer is debatable, considering that moisturizing products are not a one size fits all. The best moisturizer is the moisturizer that works best for you, based on your hair's type & condition, porosity, hairstyle, and lifestyle. The best moisturizer provides the moisture you need; it lasts all day and is compatible with your everyday styling products. In my opinion and experience, water is the best moisturizer for curly, kinky & coily hair, which is naturally dry & thirsty. Natural hair absolutely loves water, so during your natural hair care journey, you may realize that water-based moisturizers are best.

43

What are the Different Types/ Forms of Moisturizers?

There are 3 forms of moisturizers: liquid, cream, or butter/ pomade. Oil is NOT a moisturizer. Oil can be used to seal in moisture, or for hot oil scalp & hair conditioning treatments. Your hair's texture, length, and/or desired hairstyle are the determining factors of what type of moisturizer you should use. If your hair is very thick and/or coarse, you may need a butter or another kind of thick, creamy, type of moisturizer to make sure every hair strand gets the moisture it needs and retains that moisture. Thicker creams or butters may also allow natural hairstyles such as twists/twist-outs and braids/braid-outs, last longer. If your hair is thin and/or fine, a lighter product such as a liquid spray moisturizer may be best, so the hair doesn't look weighed down and limp, lacking body or volume.

44

What is a Good Moisturizing Product?

A good moisturizing product is one that hydrates the hair, reducing dryness and brittleness, setting the hair up for great styling results and softer hair.

45

What Does a Moisturizer Do?

A moisturizer does just that... moisturizes, hydrates, and softens the hair to prevent dryness, brittleness, and breakage. A moisturizer also helps keep frizz under control.

46

Can I Use Oil to Moisturize?

When you are thirsty, would you drink oil to quench your thirst?... Exactly! Then why would you use oil when your hair is thirsty and needs moisture? Oil does not moisturize hair. It can, however, be used to seal in moisture or for hot oil scalp & hair conditioning treatments, as mentioned above.

47

What is the First Ingredient a Moisturizer Should Have?

When reading a list of ingredients, always remember... 'First to Last means Most to Least.' The first ingredient in a product is the ingredient that makes up the majority of the product. With that said, water should be the first ingredient that your hair moisturizer should have, since water provides the ultimate hydration. After all, when you are thirsty, what do you drink? Water, of course!... or something that has water in it. Just look how your hair reacts to water when you first wet it down in the shower! It immediately de-frizzes and the curls clump, resulting in great hair definition and elasticity.

48

Can I Just Use Water to Moisturize?

Water, alone, can be used to moisturize the hair, but it may dissipate unless the water is combined with another ingredient that will retain moisture in the hair.

49

What Can I Do to Retain Moisture?

To retain moisture, you can seal it in with an oil, or use a product with ingredients that attract moisture to the hair. You will learn more about these ingredients and more in the ingredient section of the book. Another way to retain moisture is to sleep with a satin bonnet, satin scarf, or sleep on a satin pillowcase. Satin absorbs moisture, unlike cotton, which can suck the moisture right out of the hair!

50

How Often Should I Moisturize?

You should moisturize your hair as often as your hair tells you to. Generally, one with natural / curly hair should moisturize, on average, once a week. However, depending on hair texture, hairstyle, climate, and/or lifestyle, you may need to moisturize more or less frequently. For instance, if you live in a very humid climate, you may not need to moisturize as often as someone who lives in a dry climate. A humid climate may attract moisture to the hair, whereas a dry climate may pull moisture out of the hair and may require you to moisturize everyday (if not twice a day). Those with very porous hair may need to moisturize more frequently than others with non-porous hair, due to the hair's cuticle layer being open causing loss of moisture. If you want to have a moisturizing routine, like you may do for your skin, moisturize in the morning and at night before you go to bed... but be sure to sleep with a satin cap or on a satin pillowcase to retain moisture throughout the night.

51

Should I Moisturize Before Applying Gels, Mousses, Serums, and Other Stylers?

Some styling products may contain alcohol or other agents that may cause dryness to the hair. In this case, it's vital that you apply a moisturizer prior to applying gels, mousses, etc to avoid dryness, which can lead to breakage.

52

How Should I Moisturize Before I Straighten My Hair?

For heat styling, you may want to avoid extreme moisture to prevent reversion or frizz when trying to keep straight or curled for a certain period of time. With water being the best moisturizer (and if you prefer not to use a leave-in product), it's important to quickly blow dry damp hair to close the cuticle and lock in the moisture then heat style as you desire. For those who want extra protection, apply a light oil or heat styling product to damp hair then quickly proceed to blow dry and heat style. When straightening the hair, avoid using products that contain humectants, which attract moisture to the hair and ultimately can cause frizz and reverting.

53

What are Some Ways to Keep Hair Moisturized in Dry Conditions?

Can't stress enough that water and water-based products should be applied in abundance in drier climates just as you would apply extra moisture to your dry skin. To keep hair moisturized longer, seal the moisture in with a butter or oil. You can also do the bagging method, explained in tip number 57.

54

Why Does Natural Hair Love Water?

Natural hair is delicate, like a flower. Just like flowers, natural hair needs water to grow and flourish. Without water, natural hair will be prone to dryness, breakage, and brittleness and will wither away, just like an unwatered flower.

55

Why Isn't Oil a Moisturizer?

Generally, oils coat the hair but do not penetrate the hair shaft like water-based products can. The main reason is because the molecular structure of oil is too big to penetrate. There are, however, three common oils that actually can penetrate the hair shaft with some extra smoothing and massaging into the hair.

They are extra virgin olive oil, coconut oil, and avocado oil. Learn more about oils in Chapter 4.

56

Can You Overly Moisturize?

It is possible to overly moisturize the hair, making it look and feel limp, mushy and prone to breakage. To combat overly-moisturized hair, a protein treatment may be necessary.

57

What is the "Bagging Method?"

The Bagging Method is when you secure a plastic cap / bag over your head immediately after moisturizing the hair, to allow the moisture to soak into the hair shaft. The Bagging Method is most beneficial on the days you need extreme moisture and if you are applying drying gels or other styling products the next day, to create your defined curls.

58

Can Water Dry Your Hair Out?

Water acts as a moisturizer but, depending on the hair texture, it can be drying if you are not locking in that moisture with another product. Water alone evaporates or dissipates quickly, and could result in dry-looking and/or feeling hair.

59

What is the "LOC method?"

The Liquid, Oil, Cream method was introduced to the natural hair world by Rochelle Graham, the creator of Alikay Naturals, during her YouTube days. It's a moisturizing technique that consists of hydrating the hair with water or a water-based moisturizing spray (your liquid), sealing in the moisture with oil, then closing the hair's cuticle with a cream product to prevent moisture loss. Some also use the LCO method to moisturize and seal: Liquid, Cream, Oil.

60

How do I Know Which Form of Moisturizer to Use?

There are 3 forms of moisturizers: liquid, cream, or butter/pomade. Choosing a moisturizer depends on your hair texture, porosity, and density. A heavy moisturizing cream or butter may work for someone with very thick and coarse hair, but may be too much for someone with very thin or fine hair, weighing the hair down and making it look super limp and greasy. One may do better with a light moisturizing spray, versus a cream or butter.

4

Sealing & Oiling

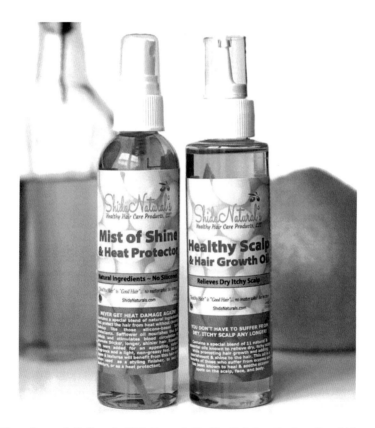

*Photo of natural oils from the ShidaNatural's Healthy Hair Care Products line which can
be used to effectively seal and/or oil hair and scalp*
www.shidanaturals.com

61

What is "Sealing?"

Sealing, in the hair world, is a term used to mean sealing in moisture. Sealing in a water-based moisturizing product allows the hair to retain moisture for a longer period of time.

62

What Can You Seal With?

The most common product that naturals seal with is generally an oil, while some use creams or butters to seal. Again, different hair textures call for different products and/or product application techniques.

63

Why is Sealing Important?

Depending on hair's porosity, sealing in moisture can be crucial if you want to prevent dry hair. Hair that has high porosity is more prone to dryness, since this type of hair doesn't seem to retain moisture for long periods of time. Dry weather conditions can also cause dryness to the hair and sealing in moisture may help keep the hair moisturized longer in this type of climate.

64

When Should You Seal?

You should seal if you feel like your hair is not retaining moisture, or if you want to add shine to it .

65

Who Needs to Seal?

Those with high porosity hair should seal not only to help retain moisture for a longer period of time, but also to add shine to the hair while closing the hair's cuticle, resulting in more shine.

66

What Are the Best Oils to Seal With?

I wouldn't necessarily say there is one oil that's the best oil to seal with. I would say the most common are extra virgin olive oil and coconut oil, but you can also seal in moisture with almond oil, avocado oil, grapeseed oil, or whatever you choose as your favorite oil to seal with. Different oils have different benefits.

67

What are the Benefits of Oiling the Hair and Scalp?

B esides sealing in moisture, oil can be used to add shine to the hair, or make it appear sleeker. Oiling the scalp has many benefits as well, like nourishing and soothing it. Certain essential oils can be added to a carrier oil, such as extra virgin olive oil or some of the other oils listed in tip number 66, to promote a healthy scalp, which can result in healthier hair growth.

68

How Can I Use Oil as a Treatment?

O il can be used in a hot treatment to improve the feel and condition of hair that is dry, brittle, and damaged. A hot oil treatment also helps replenish natural oils lost from using harsh shampoos. For best results and penetration, heat the oil before applying to damp hair, then cover with a plastic cap. For even deeper penetration, apply a wet hot towel over your plastic covered head, getting a steam treatment and hot oil treatment all in one storing!

5

Ingredients

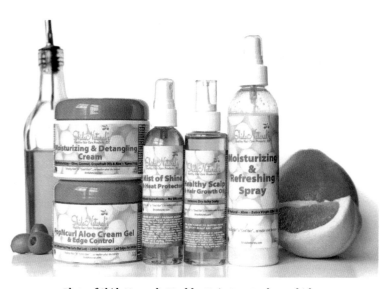

*Photo of ShidaNatural's Healthy Hair Care Products which
are made with natural ingredients*
www.shidanaturals.com

69

Is it Good to Mix Different Products Together?

Some products mix well together, some don't. For example, pairing a certain moisturizing product with a styling gel may not be a good mix. What products mix well and don't mix well are dependent on the ingredients in the products, as well as hair porosity. For those reasons, certain product combinations may not penetrate into the hair shaft but rather cause buildup on the hair with the potential, of resulting in white residue. We will make more sense of this subject in some of the other tips in this chapter. As a side note, many hair product companies formulate their products to work together as a system, and the likelihood of, for example, their moisturizing leave-in product and styling product should complement each other.

70

What to Look for in Ingredients

When reading the list of ingredients on the back label of a product, always remember, as I've said before... First to Last means Most to Least. You want to make sure the ingredients listed at the top of the list are those ingredients you can pronounce, and the added chemicals are at or near the bottom of the list. If you are one who has very dry hair, you would want to look for products that have water at the top of the list. You also want to look for ingredients that will penetrate into the hair shaft. A good way to test whether or not a product will penetrate or just sit on top of the hair is the finger test. Take a small sample of product and rub it into your fingers. If you are rubbing for a very long time and the product is not sinking into your skin, then you can almost guarantee that that product will just sit on the hair and cause product build up with frequent use.

71

What to Avoid in Ingredients

If you experience hair dryness, avoid frequent use of products (particularly in conditioners & gels) that contain certain silicones, a.k.a cones. These are those ingredients that end with "cone," "conol," or "xane." Although silicones give the hair that slick, smooth, shiny appearance, silicones coat the hair, providing a barrier that blocks out moisture. Therefore, some (not all) cone-containing products tend to cause dryness to hair with frequent use. Avoid frequent use of products (particularly in oils, cream moisturizers & pomades) that have mineral oil (aka paraffinum liquidum), petroleum, or petrolatum. Known to be used as an emollient, these ingredients may cause dryness & clog pores which may prevent the hair follicle from growing hair at its normal rate. They also do not penetrate the hair or scalp - They just sit on top of hair and scalp, which can cause product build up. If you are following the "Curly Girl Method', do not use products that contain silicones, which are explained in tip number 72.

72

What are Silicones, and How do I Know if it's a Good or Bad Silicone?

Silicones (aka cones) are those ingredients that end with "cone,» "conol,» or "xane." Silicones are found in many conditioners and leave-in products. Although they give the hair that slick, smooth, shiny appearance, some silicones coat the hair in a way that may provide a barrier that blocks out moisture. Therefore, some (but not all) cone-containing products tend to cause dryness to hair with frequent use. There are a variety of silicones that are used in different ways. Some of us may use silicones in our conditioner and/or leave-in products for the slip to aid in the detangling process and combat frizz. Others use silicones to protect their hair from heat during heat styling. Some water-soluble silicones evaporate and do not cause build-up or can simply be rinsed out without the use of a sulfate shampoo. Other non-water soluble silicones cannot be removed so easily and will require a sulfate or clarifying shampoo to remove the silicone and prevent product build up. Examples of different silicones and their categories are listed below.

Water Soluble Silicones that are easy to remove:

- Behenoxy Dimethicone
- Stearoxy Dimethicone

Non-Water Soluble Silicones that cause build up over time:

- Amodimethicone
- Cyclomethicone

- Cyclopentasiloxane
- Trimethylsilylamodimethicone

Non-Water Soluble Silicones that cause build up with each use and are hard to remove:

- Cetearyl Methicone
- Cetyl Dimethicone
- Dimethicone
- Dimethiconol
- Stearyl Dimethicone

73

What are Sulfates?

Sulfates are what provide that sudsy lather when shampooing your hair (or washing dishes). They can be very harsh and drying to the hair, especially to natural / curly hair, since their job is to strip the hair (and dishes) of all dirt, oil, and build up. In terms of hair, sulfates strip out all moisture and natural oils. If you do use a sulfate shampoo, it is recommended that you first do a pre-poo (pre-shampoo) by way of a hot oil treatment with a natural oil to make up for the loss of oils during the shampoo process. If you're going to use the no-poo/co-wash/no-cone "Curly Girl" hair regimen, prior to starting, you must first clarify hair of any build-up or cone-containing products using a sulfate shampoo. To lessen the harsh and drying effects of a sulfate shampoo, only use shampoo to cleanse the scalp on the first wash, getting underneath the hair; rinse with warm water allowing, the shampoo to gently cleanse the hair as it runs down the hair; then co-wash the hair on the second or subsequent washes.

74

Is Mineral Oil Good or Bad?

It may be a good idea to avoid or reduce frequent use of products that contain mineral oil (aka paraffinum liquidum). These ingredients are usually found in oils, creams, and pomades. Known to be used as an emollient (making combing easier), these ingredients may cause dryness & clog pores, which may prevent the hair follicle from growing hair at a normal rate. They do not penetrate the hair or scalp. They just sit on top of the hair and scalp, ultimately causing build up.

75

Is Petroleum / Petrolatum Good or Bad?

As explained tip number 74, regarding mineral oil, the same applies when it comes to the use of products containing petroleum or petrolatum.

76

Are all Alcohols Bad?

It is common to think that alcohol-containing products are not good for the hair due to the drying effects of alcohol. This is a misconception. All alcohols are not bad. There are certain alcohols that can be drying to the hair and some that are not.

The "drying" alcohols are generally found in styling products to help spread products onto the hair. They may be ok for looser curl types, as they evaporate quickly, but not ok for tighter curl types. These alcohols have different purposes, such as mixing oil and water in shampoos and conditioners, as well as helping with the absorption of hair color and other ingredients into the hair follicles.

The "nondrying" alcohols do the opposite of "drying alcohols." They actually draw moisture to the hair and provide slip, making detangling easier. These alcohols also thicken products.

The "Drying" alcohols are as follows:

- Alcohol denat.
- Benzyl alcohol
- Ethanol alcohol
- Ethyl alcohol
- Isopropanol alcohol
- Isopropyl alcohol
- Propanol alcohol

The "Non Drying" alcohols are as follows:

- Cetyl alcohol
- Cetearyl alcohol
- Stearyl alcohol
- Lauryl alcohol

As a general rule, know what you are putting in your hair then listen to your hair, as it will tell you what ingredients it can tolerate and which ingredients it cannot tolerate.

77

Should I Use All-Natural Products?

The choice to use all natural products is a personal one. Some choose to use all natural products for health, religious, or other reasons. One thing to keep in mind is that the chemicals you put in your hair and scalp don't just stay on your head. They enter your pores into your body and they also go down the drain and into the environment. All natural ingredients won't pollute your body or the environment and, with continued use of all natural products, your hair, scalp, and skin will be healthier over time. If you are not using all natural products, it's best to do your own research on what you are putting in your hair, scalp, and skin to ensure those chemicals in your products don't affect your overall health.

78

What is a Humectant?

A humectant is an ingredient added to products to attract moisture from the environment to the hair. This science helps the hair retain moisture, so the hair stays moisturized for a longer period of time. Take caution when using humectant-containing products in high humidity conditions. In these conditions, too much water can be attracted to the hair resulting in frizz and loss of curl definition. The opposite can occur in low humidity conditions where moisture will be removed from the hair, making the hair dry, but will result in less frizz. Sealing with an oil or butter may lock in that moisture and prevent dryness.

Common humectants found in hair products are as follows:

- Butylene Glycol
- Glycerin
- Honey
- Panthenol
- Propylene Glycol

79

What Ingredients Can Cause Product Build-Up on Hair and Scalp?

Review tips 70, 71, 72 and 74 to be reminded of what ingredients can cause product build-up on the hair and scalp.

80

What is the Importance of Reading the Ingredients List from First to Last?

When reading list of ingredients, always remember the mantra... First to Last means Most to Least. The first ingredient in a product is the ingredient that makes up the majority of the product. Many companies promote the natural, so-called good, or consumers' most desired ingredients on the front of their packaging. Regardless of what ingredients are being advertised on the front label of the bottle or jar, it's more important to see where those ingredients fall on the ingredients list on the back label. Are they close to the top of the list or the bottom?

81

Can I Make my Purchase Decisions by Reading Only the Front Label?

As stated in tip number 80, you should make your hair product purchase decisions based on the ingredients listed on the back label rather than the front label. The front label does not list ALL the ingredients that are in the product, but rather a few ingredients the company wants to advertise to the consumer.

82

What Ingredients Should I Avoid if My hair is Always Dry?

If you experience constant hair dryness, avoid products (particularly in conditioners, moisturizers, and gels) that have silicones. Although silicones give the hair slick, smooth, shiny appearance, silicones coat the hair providing a barrier that blocks out moisture. Therefore, silicone-containing products tend to cause dryness to hair with continued use. You should also avoid products (particularly in oils, cream moisturizers & pomades) that have mineral oil (or the fancy name, paraffinum liquidum), petroleum, or petrolatum. Known to be used as an emollient, these ingredients may cause dryness & clog pores which may prevent the hair follicle from growing hair at normal rate. They do not penetrate the hair or scalp. They just sit on top of the scalp and hair.

83

What is an Emollient?

Emollients provide slip, making detangling easier. They also smooth the hair's cuticle to reduce tangles, resulting in shine. Most common emollients in hair products are butters, oils, fatty alcohols, silicones, mineral oil, petrolatum, and polyquaterniums.

6

Hair Cutting & Styling

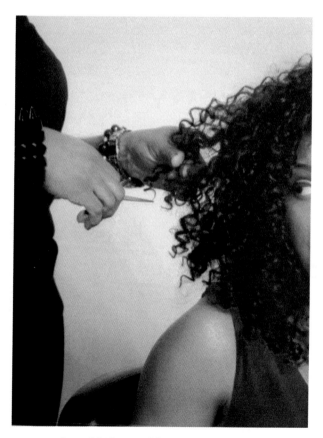

Photo of ShidaNatural demonstrating a curly cut

84

When to Cut your Natural / Curly hair

There are different reasons why we cut our natural / curly hair. You may be transitioning from chemically treated or heat damaged hair to your 100% natural hair texture and may be ready for the "Big Chop." You love your curls but may not necessarily like how they hang after being styled, so you may opt for a shaping or curly cut. Perhaps your ends look and feel raggedy, or you notice you have split ends, then you may just need a health cut or trim. Finally, you may want to switch up your look completely, so you go all out and drastically change your hairstyle with a trendy haircut!

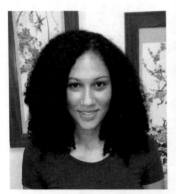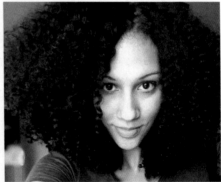

Photos of Before and After Curly Cut by ShidaNatural
Photo Credit (on the right): @taralindaaa (Instagram)

85

When to Trim Your Natural / Curly Hair

The general rule we all may be accustomed to is to trim your ends every 4 to 6 weeks, depending on your hair care and styling routine (i.e. chemicals, coloring, heat styling, excessive combing or brushing). If you don't use chemicals to permanently alter your hair's natural texture, don't color your hair, don't heat style, and/or have a low manipulation hair styling routine, it may not be necessary to trim your hair so frequently. The simple rule would then be to trim as needed.

86

What are the Different Ways to Trim your Natural / Curly Hair?

There is more than one way to trim natural / curly hair. The way you trim your ends should be dependent on how you normally style your hair, or how bad / unhealthy your ends are. A trim on blown out hair is necessary if you normally wear your natural hair straight or you need a thorough trim due to very raggedy or split ends. I never suggest trimming natural / curly hair in its wet state if you normally wear your hair curly and don't heat style. Due to the "shrinkage" factor, it is likely that when your curls dry, they will shrink to different lengths since most of us have different curl textures and patterns throughout our heads. Some curls are looser, some are tighter. Therefore, the final result of trimming natural / curly hair in its wet state will appear uneven. My personal favorite way to trim my hair is the curl by curl trim after my curls have already been defined and dried in their natural curl pattern. An uncommon but very effective way to trim natural / curly hair is the search and destroy method, where you go around your head looking for split ends and clipping the split ends... only, without cutting good hair that is not split. This is a great option for those with longer lengths. One final and super easy way to trim ends is to put your freshly detangled hair into two-strand twists, let hair air dry, then trim the tips of the twists.

87

What are the Different Ways to Cut your Natural / Curly Hair?

The different ways to "trim" hair as explained in tip number 86, can also be applied when "cutting" natural / curly hair. The only difference is you may be cutting off more length to attain a specific style or shape.

88

Wash n Go (Pop n Curl ™)

A Wash n Go (or) Pop n Curl ™ (which is what we call it at Kin-Hairitage Natural Hair Salon) is a hairstyle that's achieved with your own natural curl pattern using styling product and technique to define and lock in your natural curl pattern. The product and technique used will depend on hair texture, density, porosity, length, and desired curl definition results (super defined, mildly defined, lots of volume, little volume to no volume). Common Wash n Go styling products are gels, curl creams, mousses, and liquid serums. Common Wash n Go styling techniques are shingling (rake & smooth), finger coiling, and scrunching. Again, depending on desired styling results, some prefer to air dry while others prefer to blow dry with a diffuser to keep the curls intact.

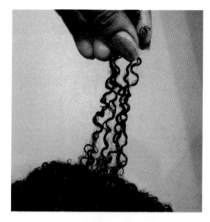

Photo of defined curls, up close and personal
Product Used: ShidaNatual's
PopNcurl Aloe Cream Gel &
Edge Control
Technique Used: Shingling
(Rake and Smooth)
www.shidanaturals.com

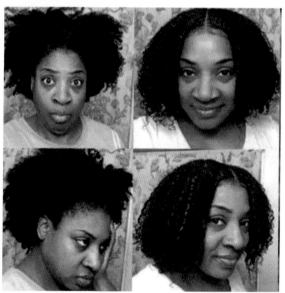

Photos of Before and After PopNcurl™ on ShidaNatural
Product Used: ShidaNatual's PopNcurl Aloe Cream Gel & Edge Control
Technique Used: Shingling (Rake and Smooth)
www.shidanaturals.com

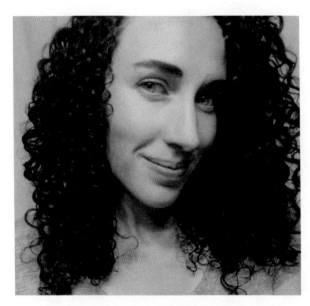

Photo of PopNcurl™ on Emily Jane
Product Used: ShidaNatual's PopNcurl Aloe Cream Gel & Edge Control
Technique Used: Rake and Scrunch **www.shidanaturals.com**
Photo Credit: @emilyjanecurls (Instagram)

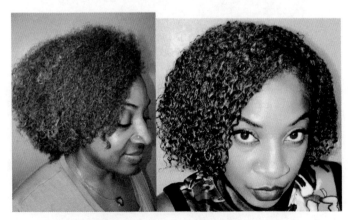

Photos of Before and After PopNcurl™ on ShidaNatural
Product Used: ShidaNatual's PopNcurl Aloe Cream Gel & Edge Control
Technique Used: Shingling (Rake and Smooth)
www.shidanaturals.com

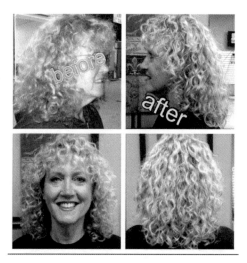

Photos of Before and After PopNcurl™ by KinHairitage Salon
Product Used: ShidaNatual's PopNcurl Aloe Cream Gel & Edge Control.
Technique Used: Rake & Scrunch
www.kinhairitage.com, www.shidanaturals.com

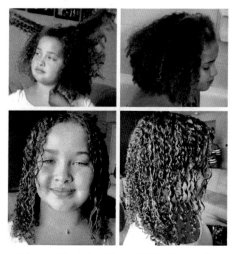

Photos of Marla's Before and After PopNcurl™
Product Used: ShidaNatual's Pop n Curl Aloe Cream Gel & Edge Control
Technique Used: Shingling (Rake and Smooth)
www.ShidaNaturals.com

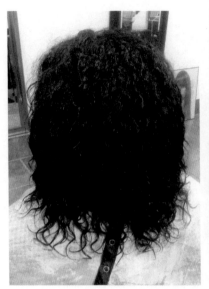 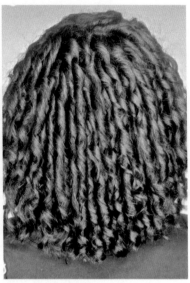

Photos of Before and After PopNcurl™ by KinHairitage Salon
Product Used: ShidaNatual's PopNcurl Aloe Cream Gel & Edge Control
Technique Used: Finger Coiling
www.kinhairitage.com
www.shidanaturals.com

89

Afro / Curly Fro

To achieve a bigger, more voluminous look like an afro / curly fro, use less styling product, a blow dryer with diffuser, and a pick.

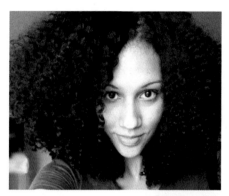

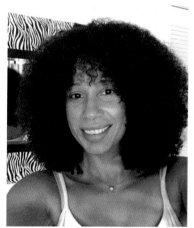 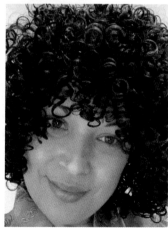

Bottom right photo of PopNcurl™
Photo Credit: @curlyqueenblue (Instagram)
Product Used: ShidaNatual's PopNcurl Aloe Cream Gel & Edge Control
www.shidanaturals.com

90

Twistout

A twistout is another style for those who like big hair. The more you separate the clumped hair strands, after unravelling the twists, the more volume you will achieve.

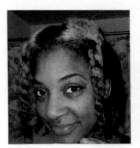
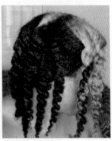
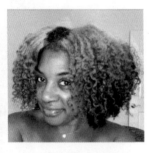

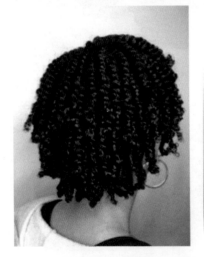
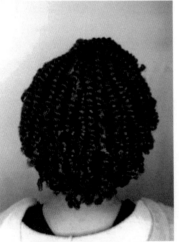

Top photos of two strand twists and twistout on ShidaNatural
Bottom photos of twistout by Kinhairitage Salon
Product Used: ShidaNatural's Moisturizing Cream & Detangler
www.kinhairitage.com, www.shidanaturals..com

91

Bantu Knots / Bantu Knotout

Bantu knots are little buns, traditionally worn by African women of different cultures. They can be worn as knots or take them down to rock a bantu knot out. When people refer to the Tracee Ellis Ross hairstyle, they most likely are referring to a bantu knot out. This is a great style for those transitioning out of a relaxer to their natural hair texture, but not quite ready to do the Big Chop.

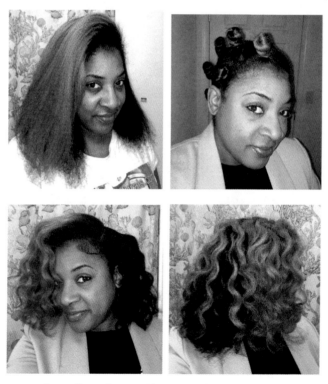

Photos of bantu knots and bantu knotout on ShidaNatural
Product Used: ShidaNatural's Moisturizing Cream & Detangler
www.shidanaturals..com

92

Braids

Want to give your hair a break from daily styling and manipulation? Then a protective style such as braids (with added hair) is the perfect way to go. Braids can be very versatile and worn in so many ways.

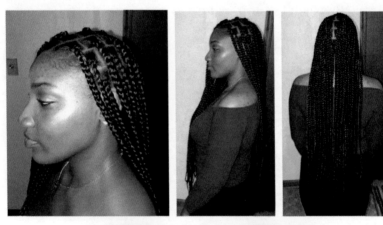

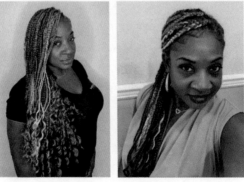

Photos of Knotless Braids by KinHairitage Salon
www.kinhairitage..com

93

Twists

Twists (with added hair) is an alternative protective style option to braids.

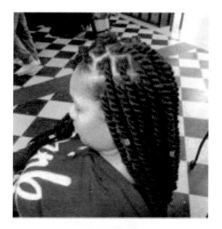

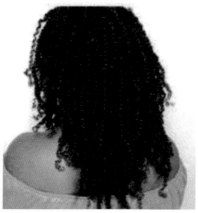

Top photo of Marley Twists by KinHairitage Salon
Product Used: MyMarlee Jam
Bottom photo of Kinetic Twists by KinHairitage Salon
www.kinhairitage.com

94

Sets (rod, flexi, straw, coils / coil-out)

A set style such as a flexirod set is an excellent choice for those with relaxed hair who desire a curly, more textured look or transitioning out of a relaxer.

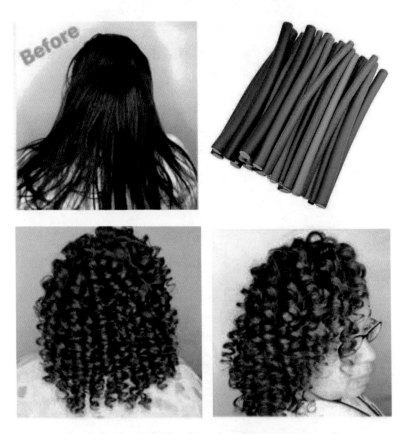

Photos of Before and After Flexirod Set by KinHairitage Salon
www.kinhairitage.com

95

Ponytails

Want a more polished look for a special occasion or just a normal day? A slicked down ponytail with your own hair or added hair is a great option. Some basic items you will need are a styling product, scarf, and, for that extra cute look, a baby hairbrush.

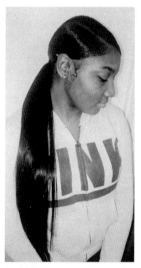

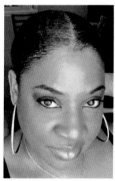
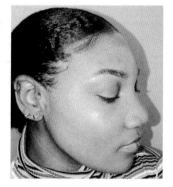

96

Banding

On days you don't want to invest too much time styling your hair, banding is a go-style for those lazy weekends, or days when you need to run errands. Banded ponytails are also a great way to stretch hair without the use of heat. All you really need are some elastic ponytail holders.

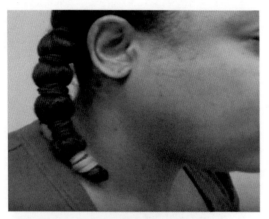

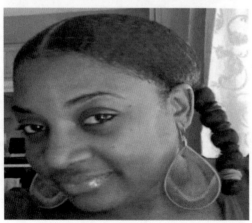

97

Bun

Bunning is also another lazy-day hairstyle, or a great one for the office. If your hair isn't long enough to fill a bun, you can always add a sock or donut to add fullness.

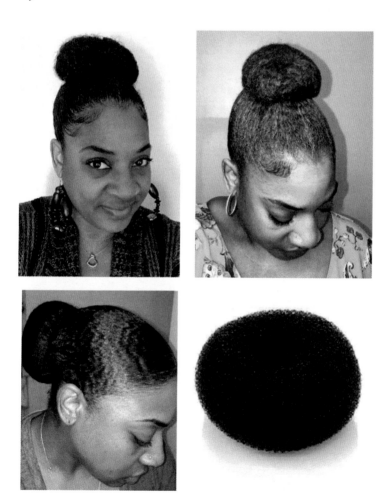

98

Updo

An updo (with added hair) is perfect for an evening out, or for when you want to make a bold statement at that special occasion and capture everyone's eyes. The twists and turns of these unique hairstyles are definitely conversation starters at any party!

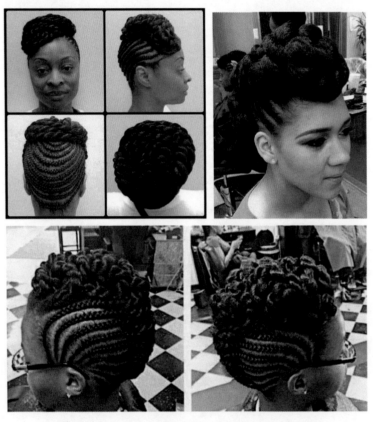

Photos of Updo styles (with added hair) by KinHairitage Salon
www.kinhairitage.com

99

Blowout / Heat Styling

If you are trying to keep your natural hair its healthiest, it's best to keep the heat away! However, we sometimes get the itch to switch it up or have some hang and flow time! If you can't resist the heat, make sure you protect your hair by using good products that will create a heat shield, and know how much heat your natural hair can take.

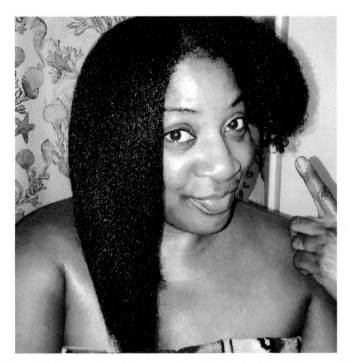

Photo of ShidaNatural and her natural curly hair after blow drying one side
"THE SHRINKAGE IS REAL!"
Products used: ShidaNatural's Mist of Shine & Heat Protector
www.shidanaturals.com

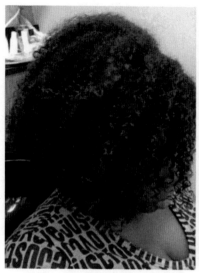
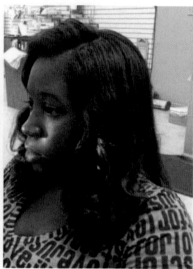

Before and After photos of a thermal press by KinHairitage Salon
Products used: ShidaNatural's Mist of Shine & Heat Protector.
www.kinhairitage.com, www.shidanaturals.com

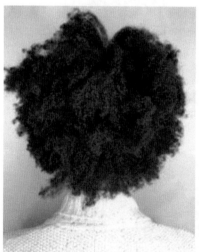
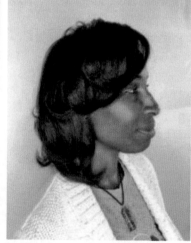

Before and After photos of a silk press by KinHairitage Salon
Products used: GREW by ME.
www.kinhairitage.com, www.mikaenglish.com

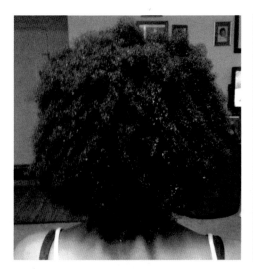
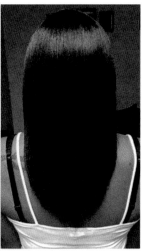

Before and After photos of a thermal press on ShidaNatural's daughter.
Products used: ShidaNatural's Mist of Shine & Heat Protector.
www.shidanaturals.com

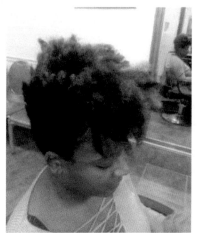
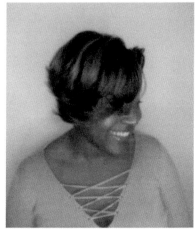

Before and After photos of a silk press by KinHairitage Salon
Products used: GREW by ME
www.kinhairitage.com
www.mikaenglish.com

100

Protective Styles

When I think of protective styling, I think about putting my hair in hibernation. Putting hair in hibernation gives your hair a break from daily styling and manipulation. Protective styling puts less stress on hair strands, especially the ends which are the most fragile. Protective Styling is a way to retain length as your hair grows while wearing wigs or hair extensions.

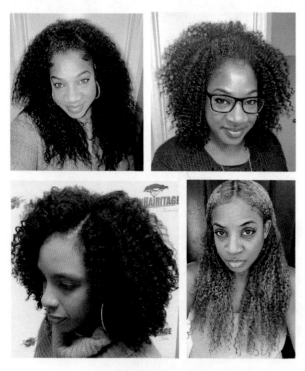

Top left photo of a half wig
Top right & bottom left photos of a catch weave installed by KinHairitage Salon
Bottom right photo of micro link hair extensions installed by KinHairitage Salon
www.kinhairitage.com

101

Locs

Locs are becoming more popular, and there are many reasons why people are making the decision to "loc up." The main reason is because locs require less maintenance on a daily basis. They are very versatile and can be styled in many different ways. If you don't want to go through the process of naturally loc'ing your hair, which requires a lot of time and patience, then permanent loc extensions may be the way to go.

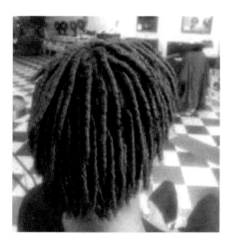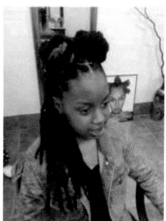

Left photo of coils / starter locs by KinHairitage Salon
<u>Product Used:</u> Nubian Kinks Pomade
Right photo of locs with buns by KinHairitage Salon
<u>Products Used:</u> ShidaNatural's Moisturizing & Refreshing Spray,
ShidaNatural's Healthy Scalp & Hair Oil, MyMarlee Jam
www.kinhairitage.com
www.shidanaturals.com

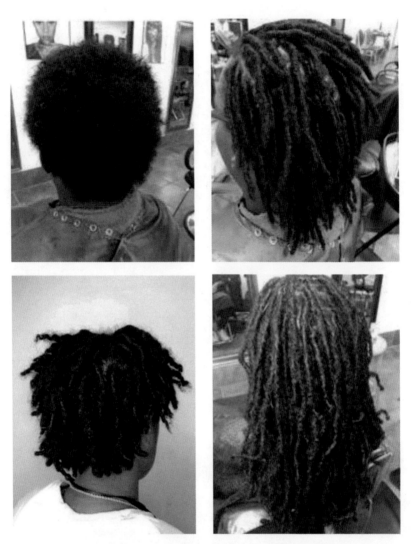

Top photos of Before & After Loc Extensions by KinHairitage Salon
Bottom photos of Before & After Loc Reattachment by KinHairitage Salon
Products Used: ShidaNatural's Moisturizing & Refreshing Spray,
ShidaNatural's Healthy Scalp & Hair Oil
www.kinhairitage.com
www.shidanaturals.com

7

Curl Talk

I had the opportunity to interview a few curlfriends about their natural / curly hair journey. They share their discoveries, successes, and challenges they faced along the way. Hopefully their stories will inspire you even more to embrace and love your natural curls.

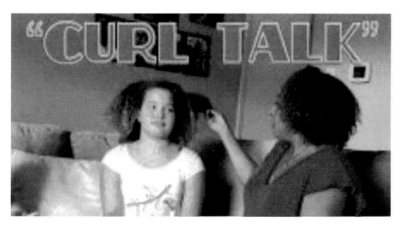

Still photo taken from an actual YouTube tutorial video of ShidaNatural's Biracial / Multiracial Curls 3-part series
www.youtube.com/shidanatural

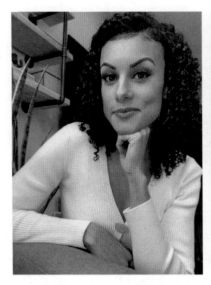
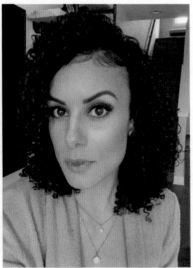

SHAINA HUMPHRIES
(Philadelphia News Anchor)
@shainahumphries (Instagram)

1. Have you always embraced your natural / curly hair?

I truly resented my hair for most of my life, until recently. When I was young, I got chemical relaxers and began flat ironing my hair. I continued to straighten and destroy my hair with heat throughout my twenties. I'm not sure specifically what inspired me to embrace my natural hair, but I certainly started to notice that more and more black and biracial women were making the decision not to conform any longer. I always just accepted my hair as something that needed to be fixed or hidden, and had never really considered that I might actually like it, or even love it, in its natural state... I just needed to learn about my texture and how to work with it. I was also growing very tired of constantly having to keep my hair straight, and I didn't really like the over-processed heat-damaged results anyway. I knew something had to change.

2. **What hair products do you use to care for and style your natural / curly hair?**

I'm always trying new products but some of my favorites so far are Kinky Curly (the Knot Today leave-in conditioner and the Curly Custard to style) and good old Cantu (the curl activator cream). I've also used some DevaCurl products here and there, but have shied away from that lately in light of some concerning headlines...

A denman brush is a key tool in the toolbox, but it creates a lot of shrinkage. It's also really important to learn how to diffuse with a blow dryer. I get better results in general by diffusing rather than air drying, plus I usually don't have the time to air dry – it takes forever!

3. **How do you usually wear your hair and why do you choose to wear it that way?**

I'm a TV news anchor and until 2020, I had always worn my hair straight on TV. Once I realized that I couldn't possibly get my curls healthy and beautiful while still straightening regularly, I started looking into wigs. Now, when I want straight hair on TV, I wear a wig. Other than that, it's usually a wash-and-go for me. It's the easiest option and I think the prettiest too – I want to see my texture in its most natural state. I sometimes throw it up into a pineapple/high ponytail look, and I'm always on the lookout for new styles that might work for me.

4. **How long did it take you to transition to fully natural / curly hair?**

Once I stopped straightening all the time, it took me several months of protective styles and trial-and-error before I felt comfortable getting a curly cut and actually going out in public. Once I went out in public, after a while I posted some natural hair pictures on social media and started talking about it publicly. A few months after that, I finally felt confident enough in the look and felt like I knew what I was doing, so I started wearing my hair natural on the air. So I would say it was about a year of experimenting before fully transitioning.

5. **What was your biggest challenge while transitioning to fully natural, and how did you overcome that challenge?**

The biggest challenge was learning how to care for and style my hair, because I had been doing it all wrong my whole life. I overcame that by sticking to it, even when it was very frustrating, watching lots of YouTube videos and following curly hair influencers on social media. Once I learned my hair type (a combination of 3b and 3c curls), I sought out information specifically for my hair type. And then, like anything, it's just practice, practice, practice. I'm 100 times better at it now than I was a few months ago, and I often really like the way my natural hair looks... And I will be even better at it a few months from now!

6. **Do you ever straighten your natural / curly hair? If yes, how do you get it straight without creating heat damage?**

At first, once I laid off the heat tools, I was still straightening with a blow dryer and flat iron once every month or so.

As I write this, I haven't straightened my hair with heat in almost 6 months. I will still straighten it a few times a year though. I love the way my hair looks straightened, now that it's healthy and LONG (let me tell you – healthy, happy hair GROWS), longer than it's ever been. But it won't look like that if I go back to frequent straightening, so it's a once-in-a-while kind of thing.

I've also been experimenting with heatless stretching techniques. The best for me so far has been Wave Formers, which I ordered online. You pull wet hair through these long, goofy-looking wavy mesh tubes. Once it's totally dry, you pull them off and have stretched, wavy, shiny hair. It's a time-consuming process and takes practice, but definitely a good option to have.

7. How often do you wash your hair?

I wash with shampoo usually once a week; I also co-wash once or twice in between. It depends on how I'm wearing my hair those days. I do a co-wash anytime I need to "reset" my curls when they've gotten frizzy after a few days, or if I'm switching from wearing a wig the day before.

8. How do you combat shrinkage?

Sometimes I just don't. It's frustrating when I see my hair, that's halfway down my back while straight, shrink up to shoulder-length when natural. But it's also a sign of healthy hair, and it's just the nature of curls. With that said, some techniques give you more shrinkage than others. I love using a denman brush to get perfectly defined, frizz-free curls. It's a game-changer for that, but – it also causes extreme shrinkage! So when I want a more elongated look,

I rake all products through with my fingers instead. It also comes out more effortless that way, with some natural curl/wave variation rather than ALL perfectly-formed spirals. There are many videos and tutorials online for those who want to learn how to apply products right and get your curls to "clump" together the way you want.

9. **How do you combat dryness and frizz?**

Water is key! I style my hair soaking wet, and I use a spray bottle mister to re-wet any sections that start to dry before I get to them with leave-in and styling product. It's also important to find the right products for your hair type, not only the wave/curl/coil pattern, but for your porosity. Water-based products work better for some, cream-based work better for others. The way you apply products also makes a huge difference. It took me months to figure out how to use both a denman brush and my fingers the right way to minimize frizz and get certain sections to clump the right way. Learning about finger-coiling is key too (though I wouldn't do that for my whole head, a denman brush achieves the same thing in much less time!)

10. **What is your nighttime routine that helps you preserve next day curls?**

The Pineapple is key! I use a loosely-wrapped satin scrunchy to gather all my hair on the very top of my head, and then either use a silk scarf or satin-lined sleep cap or bonnet, on TOP of a silk pillowcase, which is just good for everyone's hair and skin. The next day I "refresh" my hair by lightly re-wetting with a mister, using a little extra product to fix any frizzy strands, and diffuse.

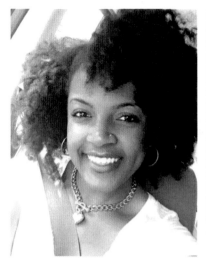 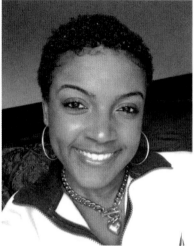

SHAWNTIA APPLEWHITE
ShidaNatural's Daughter & Keto Coach
@ketokutie_ (Instagram)

1. Have you always embraced your natural / curly hair?

No, I have not. When I turned 16, I decided to cut it off and start fresh. My mother inspired me because I saw how beautiful her curls were and how FAST her hair grew! So I wanted in!

2. What hair products do you use to care for and style your natural / curly hair?

I use ShidaNatural's cream and gel to keep my puffs secure or my twist outs popping!

3. How do you usually wear your hair and why do you choose to wear it that way?

In the fall/winter, my go-to is a twist out; but in the summer I wear protective styles, because my hair shrinks so much in the heat.

4. How long did it take you to transition to fully natural / curly hair?

One day I just had my brother take the clippers and go full force.

5. What was your biggest challenge while transitioning to fully natural and how did you overcome that challenge?

Finding decent wigs when I was bald. I was too insecure to wear my head out. I needed a little length.

6. Do you ever straighten your natural / curly hair? If yes, how do you get it straight without creating heat damage?

Yes, in the winter to get a trim and length check. I use ShidaNatural's mist of shine spray as a heat protectant. It works wonders! Never had any heat damage.

7. How often do you wash your hair?

Too embarrassed to say. Next question.

8. How do you combat shrinkage?

I do the banding method as soon as I get out the shower, let it air dry, then proceed with my twists for maximum length.

9. How do you combat dryness and frizz?

By using that Shida crack!!! I mean the ShidaNatural's cream and curl defining gel.

10. What is your nighttime routine that helps you preserve next day curls?

Large twists, ShidaNatural's oil on ends, scarf, and bonnet.

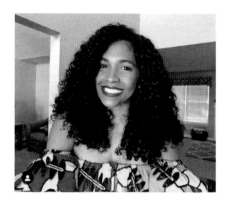 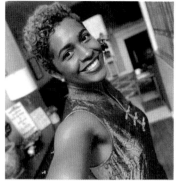

NICOLE "IvyCharlaine" BARRINGER
YouTuber
@ivycharlaine (Instagram)

1. Have you always embraced your natural / curly hair?

No I haven't always embraced my naturally curly hair. I grew up in a strict Jamaican household, and we weren't allowed to change our hair (cut/relax/flat-iron). So I wore my hair in braids, twists and buns until the 11th grade, when I rebelled and put a relaxer in my hair. I always thought that smooth, straight hair was to be desired. To be honest, anything opposite of my own natural hair was beautiful in my blinded eyes. So I relaxed and then flat-ironed my hair through college and my early 20s. It wasn't until 2010 when I started watching YouTube and saw some beautiful woman with all different types of curly and coily hair, and I was amazed. Then I noticed gorgeous naturals all around me, and it peeked my curiosity about my own hair, so I made the decision to stop straightening it and allow my curls to grow in.

2. **What hair products do you use to care for and style your natural / curly hair?**

When I find hair products that work, I tend to stay very loyal. Since the very first few years of me being natural, I've been faithfully using Kinky Curly Knot Today leave-in conditioner and ShidaNatural's Moisturizing and Detangling Cream. I alternate between the two, depending on the season and how dry my hair is. I also use different Shea Moisture rinse-out conditioners and shampoos.

3. **How do you usually wear your hair and why do you choose to wear it that way?**

I'm very low maintenance, so I tend to wear my hair in a wash 'n go the majority of the time.

4. **How long did it take you to transition to fully natural / curly hair?**

It actually took me about a year to fully transition.

5. **What was your biggest challenge while transitioning to fully natural and how did you overcome that challenge?**

My biggest challenge while transitioning to fully natural was having patience! Which was extremely hard because when I make my mind up about something, I tend to want it right away. [For] the majority of the transition, I hated how my hair looked. Every 2-3 months I got a big trim to cut away the dead, straight heat damaged ends. The cuts were not really for style, but simply to get rid of the ends. So it was very difficult for me. Twist outs and braid outs never looked nice on me, so I simply had to just wait. I kept watching other people's natural hair transition journey on

YouTube and that inspired me to keep going and not give up. It was at that time that I started documenting my journey on YouTube as well, which kept my mind off of the slow year of transitioning.

6. Do you ever straighten your natural / curly hair? If yes, how do you get it straight without creating heat damage?

I actually haven't straightened my hair in years. I don't really have the desire to straighten it anymore. I absolutely love my curls.

7. How often do you wash your hair?

I shampoo my hair probably once every 2 weeks. I normally do a co-wash or water wash twice a week.

8. How do you combat shrinkage?

I don't really do anything to combat shrinkage. In 2018, I cut off almost 20 inches of my hair into a super short curly buzz cut. In July 2019 I decided to stop cutting my hair and now I'm growing it back. I definitely have a lot of shrinkage and it looks a lot shorter than it is, but that doesn't bother me at all.

9. How do you combat dryness and frizz?

My hair definitely tends to get dry and is naturally very frizzy, especially in the cold months. During that time, I normally deep condition my hair once a week and I use ShidaNatural's Moisturizing and Detangling cream and I seal it with an oil, usually olive oil or grapeseed oil. I make sure I keep my hair extra moisturized when it's super dry.

10. What is your nighttime routine that helps you preserve next day curls?

Number one thing is that I always sleep on a satin pillowcase. My hair never touches cotton. However, when my hair was super short, there was really nothing I was able to do to preserve my curls the next day, so I would have to wet my hair every morning to get my curls looking nice. Now that it's starting to grow back, I just wear my satin bonnet and, in the morning, I put a little moisturizer on my hair and pick out my roots slightly and I'm set for the day.

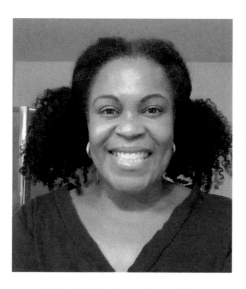

TOMMIKA BALSEIRO
Natural Hair Consultation Client
@mochabalseiro (Instagram)

1. Have you always embraced your natural / curly hair?

As you know, you were responsible for introducing me to my beautiful curls! Until that point, I felt my hair was "nappy" (I hate that word now), unruly and a burden. I feel such shame even thinking/repeating that now. My issue was that I was never taught how to properly manage my hair. It was that very reason that caused my mother to five me a perm at a very young age. I have always had "thick and long hair,"; the issue was, it always would eventually break off (due to improper maintenance). So I was always back on the journey of growing it out again. That last journey was when you introduced me to my curls, and I've been IN LOVE ever since!

2. What hair products do you use to care for and style your natural / curly hair?

I currently use Giovanni shampoo and conditioner (silk), Carol's Daughter protein deep conditioner, Shea Moisture Jamaican Black Castor Oil and kinky curly knot today for my leave-in conditioner, Shea Moisture coconut & hibiscus style milk as I am double butter cream moisturizer; Carol's daughter black vanilla combing cream— this I use for my detangler; I used a combination of different: extra virgin olive oil, grapeseed oil, sweet almond oil, avocado oil, extra-virgin olive oil. I also use rosemary, argan, eucalyptus, peppermint for essential oils. For maintenance I have a bottle that I put in my moisturizer leave in conditioners in a cup of oils and essential oils and I utilize that throughout the week to re moisturize my hair especially when it's already in a style that I want to maintain, I just spray that on my hair throughout the week make sure it gets into my strands.

3. How do you usually wear your hair and why do you choose to wear it that way?

I wear my hair in two strand twists throughout the week and wear a twist out on Sundays to go to church. This has been my process since getting into a car accident on March 25, 2015. It's the only way I can maintain it due to my physical limitations. Prior to this I would wear a wash 'n go.

4. How long did it take you to transition to fully natural / curly hair?

I would get a perm every 6 weeks (like clockwork). Eventually, my hair would start to break off and I would give it a break....cut it....wear wigs or sew-ins and then in 6 months or so....get another perm. So at the time I decided to give natural a try, I was completely perm-free.

5. **What was your biggest challenge while transitioning to fully natural and how did you overcome that challenge?**

I would like to say my challenge AFTER going natural was dealing with my hair in general. I always went to the salons, so there was a 6 month period of getting to know my hair and how to maintain it.

6. **Do you ever straighten your natural / curly hair? If yes, how do you get it straight without creating heat damage?**

No, I really don't put heat in my hair. I sweat very easily and when I do my roots are wet and there will no longer be a straight situation....my curls don't play....it's curly or nothing!!! LOL

7. **How often do you wash your hair?**

Once a month (but I may do a co-wash in between if needed).

8. **How do you combat shrinkage?**

I don't, I brace it. If there is a style that I want a little length, I will band it or stretch it by Bobby pinning my twist from one side to another.

9. **How do you combat dryness and frizz?**

My mixture of moisturizers, leave-in conditioner and oils. I spray my hair every day with water. I have a mister, or a spray bottle and I use one or the other depending on my style at the moment, then I spray on my mixture.

10. What is your nighttime routine that helps you preserve next day curls?

Depending on the style, I will wear a bonnet or a scarf. I also have a satin pillowcase that on my lazy days I will leave it out and sleep on that.

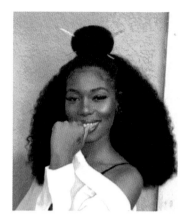 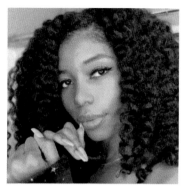

CHIME EDWARDS
OG Natural Hair Vlogger & Film Maker
@chimeedwards (Instagram)

1. Have you always embraced your natural / curly hair?

No, definitely not. The goal was to get my hair as straight as possible. It wasn't until I took an African American studies class in college did I realize how much we were changing our authentic selves to assimilate. I began to see how I was stifling my African beauty. I began to look at myself and the world differently from that point on. I began to transition the fall semester of my Senior year (2006) and graduated with 4 inches of new growth.

2. What hair products do you use to care for and style your natural / curly hair?

My top favorite products are Giovanni's Weightless Moisture leave-in conditioner, the TGIN Daily Butter Creme Moisturizer and the entire CURLS Poppin Pineapple line are everything.

3. **How do you usually wear your hair and why do you choose to wear it that way?**

I like to wear twist-outs because they're quick and easy to set and I love the results I achieve. Big, free, moisturized hair.

4. **How long did it take you to transition to fully natural / curly hair?**

I transitioned for 2 and a half years before I decided to cut the relaxer ends. I thought my head was waaaay too big for a big chop.

5. **What was your biggest challenge while transitioning to fully natural and how did you overcome that challenge?**

It was hard finding styles that looked good with my 2 textured hair - the new growth and relaxed ends. I started relaxing my edges and it made everything easier. Each style I attempted looked so much better and I could even wear my hair in a bun. I stopped relaxing my edges about 4-5 months before I cut off all my relaxed ends completely. If they had bomb edge controls like they have now back then, I could have easily avoided relaxing my edges, but it definitely was a life saver then.

6. **Do you ever straighten your natural / curly hair? If yes, how do you get it straight without creating heat damage?**

No, I haven't straightened my hair in 5 years. I really don't have the desire to. I'm deathly afraid of heat damage.

7. **How often do you wash your hair?**

I wash my hair every week and a half.

8. How do you combat shrinkage?

Honestly, I don't get very much shrinkage. My natural hair texture looks like I've blown my hair out before twisting it. I used to hate the fact that I didn't really have an actual fro like Angela Davis, but I've learned to love my hair.

9. How do you combat dryness and frizz?

I moisturize and seal daily. Using the LCO (liquid, cream and oil) method definitely has helped me eliminate dryness and a lot of frizz. My hair still will get frizzy sometimes and I've learned to accept it. I didn't go natural to have perfect hair. I wanted big, wild and free hair so I'm comfortable with letting "Diana" do her thang.

10. What is your nighttime routine that helps you preserve next day curls?

I moisturize my hair while it's in 4 sections. I dampen my hair with a vegetable glycerin and water mix (20% glycerin) then apply a leave-in conditioner, cream, and oil. Then I create one, big twist in each section and thrown on a satin bonnet. That's it! Then I'm out like a light!

8

Testimonials

It has been an honor and a privilege to have been able to help thousands of women (and men) care for, style, embrace, and fall in love with their natural / curly hair. Whether they were a Natural Hair Consultation Client, KinHairitage Salon Client, or ShidaNatural's Healthy Hair Care Products Customer, they all hold a special place in my heart. Many are not only clients or customers, but have become dear friends of mine. In this chapter, I will share with you some of their testimonials.

"Loving my hair for the first time in my life!"
"My curls are back!"
"Curls popping like crazy!"
"Curls are so defined and shiny!"
"My hair is soft and moisturized and has that shine I was looking for. My curls are poppin'!"
"My results are fabulous!"
"My curls look nice with other products but don't compare to what my curls look like with ShidaNatural's!"
"Love this stuff and so does my hair!"
"I won't use anything else on my daughter's hair!"
"My hair has never been so soft, bouncy, and shiny. This stuff is amazing!"

"Best product ever for my curls!"
*"It's so hard finding a natural product not only good for my
hair but will pop my curls and won't leave them hard!"*
"My spiralicious curls stay soft, moisturized, and touchable!"
"I'm so glad I discovered ShidaNatural!"
*"My hair is transforming and I can't believe it, soft natural
tight curls (my hair was straight up DRY Nappy)!"*
*"My eczema is not only under control but the skin
is not scaly, itchy, or painful!"*
*"My hair has improved in so many ways,
softness and growth!"*
*"Your hair care products are incredible!
My natural curl definition is amazing!"*
*I followed ShidaNatural's instructions and love how soft
and manageable my natural hair is now!"*
My hair has sheen and it hasn't in a long time!"
*"My beautiful, healthy, long, curly mane is a testament to
ShidaNatural's abilities and dedication to her hair clients."*
*"My curls are defined, shiny, soft, with movement.
I'm in love!"*

About The Author

Rashida Godbold, aka **"ShidaNatural,»** is an award-winning, recognized leader in the natural and curly hair community. Featured on Essence.com, various radio shows and popular hair & beauty blogs, ShidaNatural is an active leader, mentor and natural hair enthusiast who loves sharing her hair care knowledge via video tutorials, natural hair care seminars / hair shows / conferences and private consultations. When she is not caring for her clients' hair or running her hair care products company, ShidaNatural is a doting wife, mother, and grandmother.

Rashida has always had a passion for hair in some way, shape, or form. Born and raised in the southern part of New Jersey, Rashida received her Cosmetology license in 1993. She held the title as co-owner/operator of KinHairitage Natural Hair Salon www.KinHairitage.com, alongside her sister Victoria Shelton (Founder & CEO). Rashida conducted private and group natural hair consultations with her natural curly hair salon clients as well as local seminars. These information-packed consultations and seminars inspired her to write this book, giving her the ability to share her natural hair care knowledge with naturals all around the world.

ShidaNatural started to embrace her hair's natural texture in 2006 and, while going through her own natural hair journey, ShidaNatural started creating her own concoctions to combat those natural hair challenges many of you are familiar with. In 2008 and at the request of her hair salon clients, she launched her very own hair care product line, ShidaNatural's Healthy Hair Care Products www.ShidaNaturals.com. It became her mission to produce hair products that provided real solutions to common hair challenges, particularly those with natural curly, kinky, or coily hair!

Connect with ShidaNatural and learn more:

www.ShidaNaturals.com

www.KinHairitage.com

www.Facebook.com/ShidaNaturals

www.Facebook.com/KinHairitage

www.YouTube.com/ShidaNatural

www.Twitter.com/ShidaNatural

www.Instagram.com/ShidaNatural

www.Instagram.com/ShidaNaturals_PopNcurl